How to Dominate a Woman in Bed

Why women like to be dominated

& how to do it right

By

Lionel Maximilien

How to Dominate a Woman in Bed: Why women like to be dominated & how to do it right Copyright

ISBN: 9781973269274

Warning and Disclaimer

Every effort has been made to make this book as accurate as possible. However, no warranty or fitness is implied. The information provided is on an "as-is" basis. The author and the publisher shall have no liability or responsibility to any person or entity with respect to any loss or damages that arise from the information in this book.

Publisher Contact

Skinny Bottle Publishing

books@skinnybottle.com

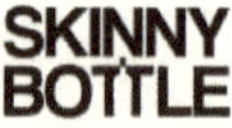

Introduction

Forget about everything you've ever read or heard that says you have to be the alpha male. Forget about those movies where the guy always gets the girl his way. And most certainly, get rid of the notion of a woman being a conquest that you are out to discover. There is far more to the secrets of learning how to dominate a woman in bed. Let me tell you right away that if you think you are going to learn how to dominate a woman out of a book you are fooled.

There is no way to logically ever figure a woman, or any person out. You have to get out there and have hands-on experience, you have to meet the right one for you and really tune in to what makes that individual tick.

What you will get from this book, is some insight in to some of the mysterious ways that combine seduction, examples and tips on domination, and a reminder of what it means to be a man in the bedroom. It's elusive and tricky, to say the least, and when you get there, you will know it. There is a little bit of psychology (okay a lot) that you will have to understand.

There is a sociological aspect to the role that men like to be the pack leader, the head of the pyramid, the king, the lion of the jungle, the knight in shining armor. You get the drift. There isn't anything wrong with this by any means. But you will find that some men like to announce their position of power. Power could be sexual, financial, career, social. It is somewhere, somehow important to them. They will tell you that you need to keep your woman in check, that you need to let her know when she is out of place.

These things might have worked at one time when the modern woman did not exist. But women today are smart, confident, bold, aggressive just like men. This doesn't mean that they still don't want to be dominated in the bedroom. They still want this! Remember this and use it to your advantage. It's sort of the holy grail when it comes to sexually satisfying women. But learning to redefine what the word 'dominate' means and how you get to the point of doing it will most likely take a little reworking of some of the stereotypes, some of the language, and most certainly some of the cardinal approaches to getting to the point where you really are the lion roaring on top of his lioness.

Chapter 1

Dominate Before the Boudoir

The Gentleman Butler

Pleasing a woman and keeping her happy by always making sure that you are doing the right thing in her eyes, will leave you looking like a servant that is just there to take care of her. For many men, myself included, we were raised to respect woman and to listen to them, giving into whatever they may require from us. It was as if the purpose of being a man centered around making sure that the experience of control and pleasure translated over to the woman at all cost and in all areas of life. The man works all day so the wife can stay home, the man understands when the girl isn't 'in the mood', the man takes care to listen to incessant rambling even when he'd rather just watch the game. Now don't get me wrong, there is a certain important truth in treating a woman with absolute respect and dignity, but that does not make you her butler or servant.

Why You're Silver Plating

When you do something nice for her you have to specifically let her know why you are doing it. Don't just give her flowers, take her out to dinner, and ask her how she feels, without telling her that you are doing it because she is yours. You have to have your moment where you redefine that the whole reason that you are giving into her and doing all those things that make her smile aren't just because she's a beautiful goddess that you want to worship.

Those might be nice gushy words that you really want to say with all of your heart, but you have to tone that down, and start to settle with what makes more sense, and that's to listen to your true desire to be dominant.

Give her nice things, treat her like the goddess that you know she is, but stand up a bit and remember that you are also a God in her eyes. Let her know that the flowers are because she is 'your favorite girl' not 'just because'. This lets her know that you have some sexual prowess by putting the notion in her head that there may be another woman that you are interested in, and at the very least it lets her know that there have been in the past. Regardless, the bottom line is it makes her feel special, wanted and lets her know a very important thing: that there is competition.

Eat it Up

When you take her out to dinner do something a little absurd from time to time. Order for her. Feed her. Eat her food. You're paying for it so why not take the lion's share if you want it? But don't be an ass. Don't grab an absurd large bite of her food and leave her with nothing. But don't nibble and be shy.

The point is just to subtly - there's that keyword - subtly let her know that you are the dominant one. This way when you do get back to the bedroom and you want to show her your real dominance, you have already set the stage for it. Have her eating out of the palm of your hand long before you have her back in the bedroom, or wherever the two of you decide it's time for you to peacock your dominance.

Think Service-Not Servant

You want to let her know that you are there for her, to help protect her, and also to give her the *service* that she does deserve. You don't have to make her earn it. She doesn't have to do to your every single whim and wish before your willing to dish out a little fair respect in return. That just doesn't make any sort of respectable sense.

But you do need to keep an eye out for the moments that you do something for her and she starts to act entitled to them. Trust me she is doing the same for you, and we all know that people, no matter whether you are a man or woman, like to start to toy with games when it comes to this. She may sit and try to withhold sexual favors, or even simple respect for you if she feels you aren't meeting up with her 'diva'-like status.

She wants to be put up on a pedestal and may feel that she can boss you around. You have to put this sort of behavior right in its place. Nip it in the bud. You don't have to over-react to it. But if she does something so simple as get on you for why you were five minutes late, you need to think about it in terms of this: she is upset you are five minutes late because her mind was going wild thinking of the reasons why you were. She didn't understand why you weren't there already waiting on her. The ball is really in your court already. Instead of looking at her like she is nagging, realize that she is already letting you know that she needs you. Yep, it's a sort of backwards way of doing it, but you have to read between the lines sometimes.

Because It Shows You Provide

Why is the service aspect so important? Yes, it does go beyond just being kind. It actually has a lot to do with that sort of primitive mentality that goes back to the beginning of our hunter and gatherer days. Even then we provided for each other. It's never just one-sided. So if you remind her that you are there to help provide for her, whether it's you opening the door for her, or simply giving her a shoulder to lean on she is going to bond more deeply with you.

There's a common misconception that in order to dominate a woman in bed you have to be aggressive with her everywhere else you go. You don't have to be aggressive you simply have to show her that you can stand on your own two feet and at the same time sweep her off of hers. Without asking for permission. Asking for permission is a game killer. It's the same way if you are asking her for stuff all the time. You begin to seem needy.

No woman, no matter how much she tells you it isn't a big deal, likes to be the one paying for everything and driving you around. Even if it doesn't bother her in the beginning, it starts to wear down on her image of you at being able to provide, and if you can't provide for yourself, how are you ever going to be able to take care of her wild desires in the bedroom? That is what she will eventually question too.

The good news is that most women don't really care about how big your bank account is so long as you are able to take care of your bills without asking for help from mommy. The same with your car. Having an old piece of junk of a car might not be the sexiest hot rod for a stallion like yourself to be driving but it doesn't mean you still can't drive her wild in bed. Don't be ashamed of the status of the material possessions in your life.

But if you are in the moocher phase of life, you aren't ever going to dominate a woman in bed until you get up out of bed and get busy working. Sounds harsh, but it's the way it is. You'll find it feels awesome being able to take a woman out, in your own vehicle, to a restaurant and tell her she can have whatever she wants off the menu. Then later, when the two of you get back to your own house, not hers, not your parent's, she's in your lair. Seduction has already begun. Your establishing dominance long before getting romantic. Step one.

Chapter 2

Getting Big in It

Show and Tell

When you're in the bed and you're ready to start showing her your dominance you have to step up your game and be in control. You're in the driver's seat now and it's time you drive her like a Ferrari even if she is a common sedan. The best way to take control of this is to know what you want, and if you don't know what you want then you have to fake it for a while. Watch a few pornos if you need to get educated.

For most men, it's easier to just go with the raw feeling of it. Your body will tell you what it wants. Give into it, and know that at this moment while she is with you in front of you naked, she is there to serve you pleasure. Not in the sense that her sole purpose is to please you, nothing that absurd, but you have to let go of your concerns about her pleasure a little bit in order to get in there and start giving her what she wants.

This is not the time to act like you don't know what you are doing. You have to man up and go for it. But no matter what you do you can't forget about the fact that she is there too. By that, I mean that the pleasure isn't all about you. But we will get to that a little later on. For now, you need to focus on showing her what you want and then telling her when she does it right. Show her by taking control physically. Lift her knees up the way you want them, push her hips down the way you like, and tell her, "Like this." Then tell her she's doing a good job.

Grit and Grab

The great thing about sex is that it crosses over all language barriers. You don't have to speak the same language one little bit to know that the person you are with is into it. So if she is rocking it out and you're really into it you don't have to say something stupid like, "Who's your Daddy?" Just moan a little. Get in close to her ear and growl a little. You shouldn't have to try to think about it. Just remember that if you are in close to her ear you don't want to blow her eardrum out. If you have to howl a little, just pull back from her head a bit and let out your inner wolf. Sex is very animal.

Sure some people will carry on about all this tantric, metaphysical connection of two spirits, and that is as great and wonderful as Santa Claus. For the rest of us, when we have sex it's raw, it's dirty, and very, very base and animal. Let yourself go. That's one of the great things of intimacy. So take position as the man, and let your wolf out of the shadows. She'll let you know if she needs you to stop. If she does, then you back off a little. Don't be pushy, don't act hurt or whiny about it. Just get up, walk into the other room and chill out. Be a man about it. If you need to, go hop in the shower. Odds are she'll be wanting you in less than an hour. If not, then you really need to think about finding another woman to dominate. You need to be yourself. She might have some hang ups she needs to work out. That's her problem. Not yours.

Handcuffs and Straps

Showing off your dominance is sometimes more a matter of suggestion than talk. Women are really good at picking up details. Especially when those details are a pair of handcuffs over by your nightstand or dangling off your bedpost. You don't even have to ever have used them and her mind will be reeling with delight as she wonders what you do with them, and what you might do to her if she had them on.

They don't even have to be right out in plain sight. Leave them somewhere else that she will see them, and if you really want to bring in the dominance, you need to have more than one pair. Can you really think of a time where just one pair of handcuffs were used in the bedroom? Possibly, but 2-4 is a pretty standard issue for some light BDSM.

Just realize that she's liable to want you to use them on her if you never have before and you're not quite sure how to go about, just remember to blindfold her first. Then she doesn't have to see you fumbling around. No matter what don't hesitate. Toss her down on the bed on her stomach. Blindfold her from behind. Roll her over, handcuff her to the bed and get to work doing what you do best. Dominating her.

The Talk

A lot of guys get all worked up about what to say when it comes to dirty talk. Dudes just don't really always want a talk. It's pretty simple what guys are thinking. So when it comes time to dominating her with your language let her know what you like. Tell her you love it. Tell her to do something. Don't' ask her, don't be shy about it. Start small. Don't tell her just to go down on you right away. She probably won't be into it right away. Unless your one lucky guy. But tell her to do something like take your shoes off you. Don't say the words: need, please, will you, can I. The only time you should be asking her questions in bed is when you ask her where she wants your cock. Tell her to get on her knees and make her wait for it as you taunt her.

If you start calling her dirty names, which a lot of people like, don't call her a little slut or a little bitch. Make sure you call her *your* little slut or bitch. You want to show possession when you say it so that she knows who's on top and in control, and also so that she knows that you are aroused by it. There's a big difference between name calling her a slut and telling her "You're *my* slut".

The tricky thing, and very fun playful thing, about wording, is that you can get away with saying just about anything in the bedroom as long as you say it with determination and action words. Don't ask for any sort of permission, give her very little option unless each option proves to work in your favor, and don't ever neglect to let her know whose property she is. Property in the bedroom that is. As much as woman don't like to be objectified and dominated, when it comes down to it, they want to know that they are the object of our affection and that we are the strong dominator in the relationship. Don't be afraid to remind her from time to time. Dominating is not being a dick-bag, so keep yourself in check, and she'll keep coming back.

Chapter 3

The Game

Ticking Time Bomb

She's going to test you at one point or another. The pressure that lovers have to bounce back and forth as to who is actually in control happens whether you are having a quick one-night stand or in a 6-year marriage. Especially if you are in a marriage, or a long-term relationship you know what it is like to deal with the ticking time dual power bomb as she tries to see how far you will go to prove that you are the dominant one.

To play this game or not is really all about how she goes about testing you. If she is belittling you, making you feel disrespected, or is being withdrawn about pleasing you then sorry bub but you might have to rethink this one. Power games should be more enjoyable than not. You will know when she is testing you and when she throws something out that just isn't cool, walk away. The more you feed the bear the more it will keep coming back to camp. No matter the power struggle sometimes you have to let her think she wins. Just simply remind her who is in charge next time you are in the bedroom. Be a little extra forceful. Nothing that isn't consensual, but show her who the boss is. You know how to do it. One way or another she's eventually going to blow, you just want to make sure that instead of her blowing up, it's you she ends up blowing.

Give It to Her

Giving in and giving her what she wants does not make you a lesser man, or make you less dominant. Let me say that again: It does not make you less dominant. She might be getting bossy about something she wants you to do for her that you don't want to do, but you do have to know when to pick your battles if you are in that happy little make-believe-land of love. However before you do what she's asking you to, make her say something like "Please master". Remind her. If she screams at you to go do it anyhow, just stand there with your arms crossed. You have to stand your ground. But if she does say *please master*, even sarcastically, then you have to go do it. You set the rule, she obeyed, now follow through. She will respect you more for this, even if she jokes about it than she would if you just got up like a zombie and followed her orders.

Be sure that it is you making the orders. This is what will lead to your ability to dominate her in the bedroom. If she's been wanting something new or places a special demand, then make her earn a little. This doesn't mean that she has to give you oral sex just because she asked you to pick up some milk on the way home from work, but it is an opportunity for you to shower her with your dominance. You have to play the game. When you get home with the milk, dangle it over her a little. Thank her for cooking for you, but tell you've got what she needs. Make her tell you to give it to her. Play around with this. Have fun. You'll get a feel for it.

But if she is in a funk and had a bad day and asks you rudely if you have the milk, don't just put it on the counter and walk away. Thank her again for making dinner, walk over to her and firmly put your hand on her hip and tell her she's the most beautiful woman you've seen all day. Kiss her on the neck. Walk away. Remember you just got home from work. Keep your dominance. She will be thinking what a lucky woman she is that you stopped on your way back and got her what she wanted. You might want to go see if you can help make dinner too. After all, this is no longer the stone age. Men help in the kitchen too. Cooking is sexy.

One More Time

One of the hottest things about playing this little dominance game over and over is that it never gets old no matter how long you are with somebody. Even though your days might be full of routine you can get the old cycle of establishing dominance rolling one more time so that you both get to feel the awesome roles in the relationship that you both have established. As time goes on you might think that sex has to get old but it doesn't have to if you keep everything else that goes on when you aren't having sex anything but boring. Leave her little notes when she puts her shoes on that say, "Tonight you're mine." Or when she goes to get her morning cup of coffee, take away the coffee the night before and leave another note saying that if she wants her cup of joe she has to come have her morning drink of you first.

You can play with this, and while notes may seem like the last way that you would have dominance over somebody you have to remember that remaining in the state of dominance isn't just about gagging, bondage, and slave play. It's as much psychological and emotional, and beyond anything else it should be playful. If it's not playful than you've missed part of the mark. You have to keep her happy. Dominate her all you want, but she is an independent woman. She doesn't need you nearly as much as you think. So stay playful, but aggressive. Imagine somebody taking away the coffee in the morning and wanting sex in return, she's going to be a hornet's nest when she comes in the room. Be sure you have the morning cup of you ready and brewed for her to finish off.

Chapter 4

Who's It Really For?

Be Dominant for Her Not You

While you are on your journey of learning the different ways to dominate your woman or any woman for that matter, you have to remember that even though woman do *want* to be dominated, they only want to be because it serves them in return too. Women like pleasing men and they like it when a man knows what he wants.

If you treat her right in return for all the pleasing she gives you, you will find that your confidence and swagger will soar in ways that you've never even known. That's one of the most amazing things about having a woman that you can dominate. There might be ways that you haven't even thought of dominating her and the tricky thing about it is that it would ruin it if she has to spell it out for you. So you have to push it a little, then reel it back in. Play the cat and mouse game with her keeping her forever in question as to whether or not you are the dominant type or the needy type. Just when she thinks that you're starting to go soft (emotionally) show her how in control you really are.

There's an art of seduction to this because a woman is equally dealing with her contradictory desires of wanting to nurture vs. being completely controlled and dominated. So when you give her the chance to nurture you a little, and then show her that you're really still in charge of yourself, you let her get drawn in even more emotionally which only leads to sweeten the pickings when it comes your time to shake down her tree.

Give Her a Chance to Be the Dominant One

What? Let her be the dominant one? Won't that take away from your chance of ever regaining your reign as the big man in the house? Absolutely not. Remember your *giving* her control. You're not letting her control you, there is a difference. One of the best things about switching up roles a little is that you can see some of the ways she may want to be treated. You can also get her to open up a little bit more in the bedroom if she is shy by letting her have control of the reigns.

Have her tie you up for once, let her go ahead and whip you a little or something. Tell her how to do it, boss her around. Tell her to give it to you like she wishes you'd give it to her. Then have her untie you and tell her it's her turn. Tell her that because she was such a bad dominant one you're going to have to show her how to be a master now. Tell her she can't come until you let her. Ask her if she knows how to moan like this (then make a special moaning sound) when she says yes, put a gag in her mouth. Show her how to spank. Fast, then slow, then show her the rhythm you like. Giving her the little bit of experience of dominance and then taking it back from her will have both of you fighting off from orgasm and leave the ball clearly in your court as headmaster.

Chapter 5

Focus All In Her (or On Her, It's your Choice)

The Sweet of It

Dominating a woman in bed can be a sweet soft act too. You can tell her that she needs to take all her clothes off. When she asks why, scold her gently for even asking you why, then blindfold her with a scarf and lead her into the bathroom where you have already poured her a nice hot bath with candle lights, rose petals, and even some light music that is romantic. Tell her that you know she's been really dirty lately and you're going to clean her up. Grab her by the hips really good and tell her you're going to have all of her tonight, then lead her into the bathtub.

Be careful that you help her. If you can, pick her up and just put her in the tub, you are her strong man remember? She is your little slut princess. Now take the time to actually bathe her. Use a favorite soap of hers, or better yet put a little forethought into it and get her something new that she has never had before, the new smell will set her senses on edge as she tries to figure out what it is.

Now, would be a good time to start putting some of that candle wax to use. You can pour a little across her chest and nipples. Be smart though that if you have had the candles burning for quite a while sometimes the wax can get sort of extra hot and actually feel less pleasant and more painful. Also, it's probably a good idea to have already toyed around with a little light slapping, biting, and scratching to see how well she handles a little bit of pain. Hot wax is pretty mild, as long as you haven't been burning the candles for hours.

Reward her after pouring some wax on her by giving her a strawberry. Have some ice cubes handy, the mixture of ice and the hot bath will bring her senses to a wild mixture. She won't know what to expect from you next. She's all yours. Have some fun. Keep it fun, but be firm.

Turn Up Your Animal Radio

After arriving home from work, but before taking off your monkey suit, find some music that turns you on, not her. Find something that has a beat you really want to give it to her with. Crank it up loud. Don't say a word to her, just grab her by the wrists, take off your tie and wrap it around them. Lead her over to a kitchen chair. Tie her to it like she was your pet.

Pat her on the head and tell her she's your good little bitch and that she's a good girl. Without taking your clothes off begin to rub your crotch against her mouth. Tell her you have something really good for her. Then step back a little. Maybe spank her on the ass a little. Start taking off your dress shirt. Then go ahead and let her have a taste of what you want to give her, but then pull back and put it back in your pants.

While she's still tied up to the kitchen chair go ahead and make sure that you have easy access to her before you untie her. Once you untie her you can go ahead and lead her up to the bedroom. If you have a bedroom that is upstairs all the better. Make her crawl on her hands and knees in front of you. Making her stop every once in a while mid-step. If she turns to look back at you pull on the leash and remind her to look the other way. Scold her. Then press yourself against her from behind. Let her feel your hardness. Tell her you've been waiting all day to take your pretty little bitch for a walk. When you get to the top of the stairs, don't lead her into the bedroom where she is expecting you to take her. Take her somewhere else. A spare room, a den, surprise her. Tie her to a doorknob if you have to. Make the most of your surroundings. Then ravage her like the animal that you are. You know she wants it. Make her deserve it.

Conclusion

Learning to dominate a woman in bed requires just a few basic things from you. The first is that you never ask her for permission. You never hesitate with what you want from her, and you always remind her that she is yours. The bedroom isn't the only place to dominate her, though, you have to do a little bit of it in other places in your life to keep your game up. Sure you can let her feel like she has control every once in a while, but a woman doesn't just want a man that is going to turn up the heat when they are in the bedroom and then be a dull flame when they are everywhere else. She needs him to be the swagger in every room that they are in.

She really does want him to open doors for her and she really needs him to still be that hunter that goes out (metaphorically at that) into the world to claim for himself. If you are able to show her that you are the boss of your own domain and ruler of your own kingdom, then you have given her something to be proud of.

Once you have established all of the ground rules for what you both like in terms of pleasure and pain you can go ahead and push the boundaries a little bit further and then pull them back. The cat and mouse game has to go on a little bit in terms of pleasure in pain in order for it to be something that is enjoyable for her. As a guy, you'd rather get right to the meat of it, but the woman needs a little story, a little something to fantasize about, make her not know what's coming next from you when you take total control of the situation and show her how submissive she is to you.

Remember that even though she may like to please you that it is not her role in life. She is doing it by choice and you always need to be respectful of the woman in your life that is on her knees treating you like the master that you are to her. If you give her plenty of rewards, not just materially, but emotionally fulfilling her needs, she will be loyal to you until the end.

Over time she will try to test how strong you are, she'll want to see if you truly are the man that you claim to be while you have her tied to the bed. Don't play into these drama games of hers as she is just really trying to push your buttons to see if you are still the dominant one. The more you allow the little buttons she pushes to get under your skin the closer you are to giving up little pieces of that role as master. Remember nobody had to give you the role of master. You're a man. You're a natural born master.

You are the ruler of your kingdom and you were born to be so. Just like you were born to have wild and rough sex full of heavy moaning, biting, and sweaty dripping flesh pounding on flesh. Show her that this is what it's like to be with a man like yourself. Don't let her think of you as any other way. Then when you need to, give her a little bit of control in the bedroom. Show her a taste of the sweet life. Then rip it right back out of her mouth before she gets too much of it. It's your world remember? Your house. Your rules. Your woman.

But do remember, that she can walk out anytime she likes. She isn't your slave. So be nice, be sweet about being the dominant member of the household. You don't have to be an asshole to be the macho man that your woman is dreaming of. Be nice to others when you're in public, show her that you are calm and in control wherever you go. Save all the savagery for when you're tearing her sweet body up in the bedroom.

She'll respect you even more if she sees that you are king without having to boast about it. Lots of men forget this. But acting like a big man on campus when you're out won't make her like you anymore. It'll just make you look stupid. And remember, she's a woman in the end. She really does have all the say. Never push her too far, if she is uncomfortable stop what you're doing and give it time, comfort her when she needs it. She needs you to be soft and hard, and totally, always 100% confident and in control. That's how you dominate a woman in bed.

[page intentionally left blank]

www.ingramcontent.com/pod-product-compliance
Lightning Source LLC
Chambersburg PA
CBHW051428250726
48655CB00003B/1287

* 9 7 8 1 9 7 3 2 6 9 2 7 4 *